Healing Views

*The Source of Your Suffering is Closer
Than You Think*

By

Ehab Fattal, MA

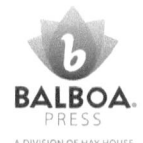

BALBOA.
PRESS
A DIVISION OF HAY HOUSE

ISBN: 978-1-4525-4737-4 (sc)
ISBN: 978-1-4525-4738-1 (e)

Balboa Press books may be ordered through booksellers or by contacting:

Balboa Press
A Division of Hay House
1663 Liberty Drive
Bloomington, IN 47403
www.balboapress.com
1-(877) 407-4847

Because of the dynamic nature of the Internet, any web addresses or
links contained in this book may have changed since publication and
may no longer be valid. The views expressed in this work are solely those
of the author and do not necessarily reflect the views of the publisher,
and the publisher hereby disclaims any responsibility for them.

The author of this book does not dispense medical advice or prescribe the use
of any technique as a form of treatment for physical, emotional, or medical
problems without the advice of a physician, either directly or indirectly. The
intent of the author is only to offer information of a general nature to help
you in your quest for emotional and spiritual well-being. In the event you use
any of the information in this book for yourself, which is your constitutional
right, the author and the publisher assume no responsibility for your actions.

Any people depicted in stock imagery provided by Thinkstock are models,
and such images are being used for illustrative purposes only.
Certain stock imagery © Thinkstock.

Printed in the United States of America

Balboa Press rev. date:11/14/2012

For Luc

The Views

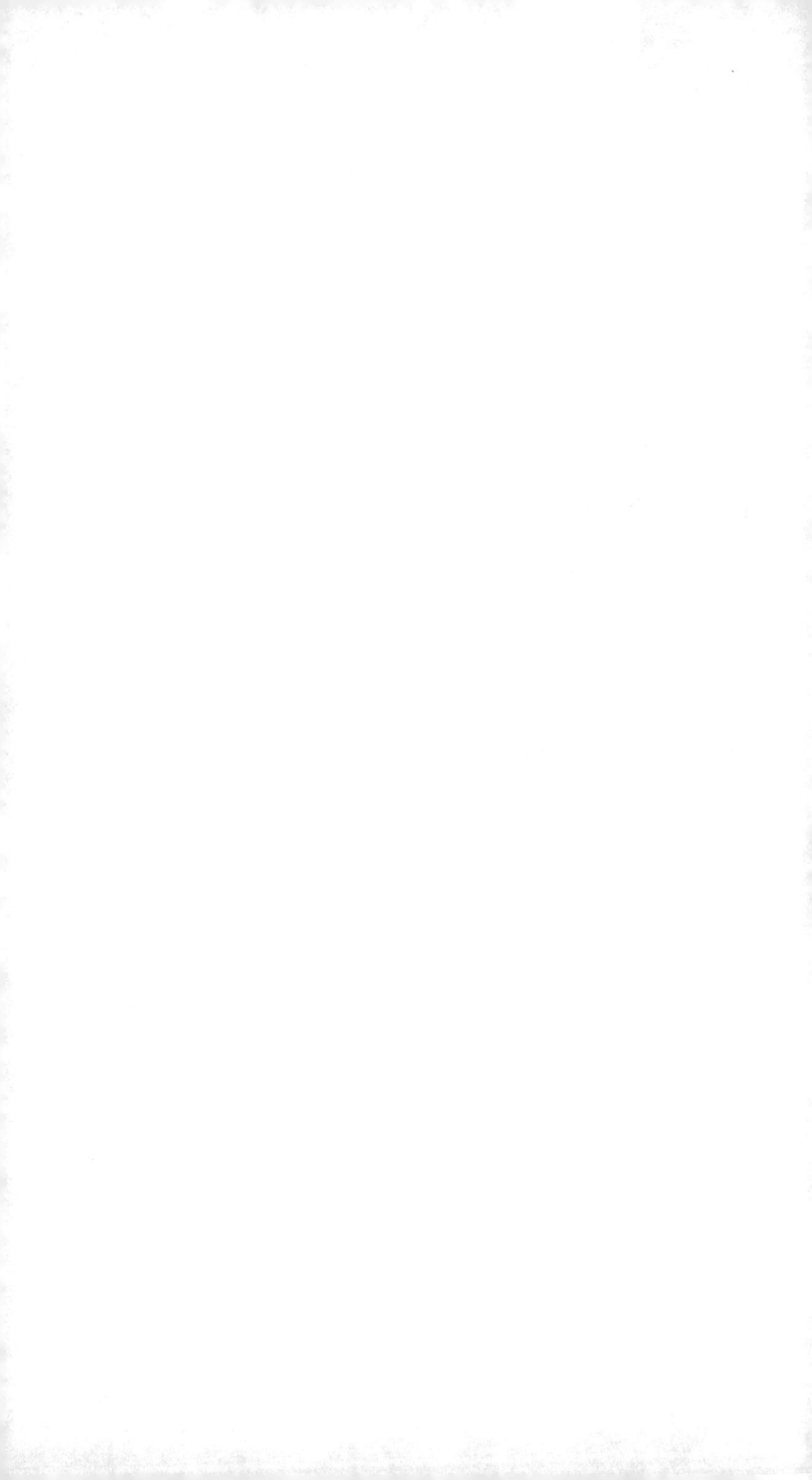

Intro

This book was written to share many of the lessons I learned that were the result of my personal struggles and experiences. Life is just one giant classroom where lessons; often harsh, lead to maturity and better understanding. All suffering, therefore, is a blessing in disguise.

Our suffering, however, may be the product of bad decision-making and lack of self-honesty. Surprisingly, most people with problems cannot admit that they actually do have a problem. Many seem to think that it is the person next door with the issues, but never them. They also contend that harsh consequences will always evade them as they insist on not changing their unhealthy lifestyle.

Although sense is fairly "common", very few choose to use it. Most burden their lives with complications; somehow feeling that they may not have a choice in the matter. We do have choices. All of us do.

This book will not solve all of your problems, but what it will do is make you aware of a different perspective on how to approach things from a more logical standpoint. Ultimately, logic is also not the only answer; people need a good balance with emotions. Finding balance is what will make you attain inner peace. Inner peace will stop your suffering and happiness will become easier to grasp.

I

Purpose

1. We are here to create and help expand the universe. That's how we worship the Creator.

   Finding out where we fit into the giant mosaic of life and pursuing it is fulfilling our life purpose. We were all born with certain skills and attributes to serve a specific function while on earth. Only when we come into full submission with who we are and what we are here to do; is when we attain inner peace and happiness.

2. Obstacles are illusions the ego creates to derail our path towards glory.

   Only those who are strong enough to withstand the power of petty distractions will reach their goal. Obstacles are not real unless we make them so. Stay focused on your final destination and all hurdles will evaporate at the snap of your fingers.

3. Try asking the question; you'd be surprised how many answers you will receive.

    We all have more power than we think. Our lack of faith is what blocks us. All of our answers are within. All we need to do is ask the question and answers will appear before us. Meditation is a very useful exercise.

4. Identify your life purpose by being true to yourself

    Self-honesty is what leads us to correct many of the imbalances in our lives. By being honest with ourselves about our capabilities and limitations is when we search for what is right for us; instead of wasting our resources on what is wrong. Your life purpose is your final destination. Pursue it and you will discover your own paradise.

5. Surrender and fly, or control and suffer.

    We are spiritual beings experiencing life. Only when we allow our spirit to call the shots instead of rely on our five senses is when we find peace. Let your spirit guide you and do not be fooled by the illusions of controlling events in your life. The spirit is much more powerful than material gains.

6. If it flows, it is natural. If it doesn't, it is time to change direction.

    The universe hinges on the delicate balance between negative and positive forces. If we encounter too much negativity while pursuing a certain path, then it is the Universe's way of telling us that it does not serve our highest good. Only when it is rightfully and naturally our true path is when all challenges are easily surmountable signaling for us to stay the course.

7. Not all roads directly lead to Rome.

    When our final destination is set and we
    are clear in our resolve on reaching it,
    some resources may become unavailable
    to help us due to the need for much
    better ones to manifest and take us to
    the next level up.

8. It is not about getting rich. It is about
    being fulfilled.

    It is impossible for everyone to be rich
    just as it impossible for everyone to
    be poor. Not everyone is an engineer
    or nurse. The diversity of functions is
    what makes life efficient according to
    the grand design. Accept who you are
    and which role you came to earth to fill
    and joy will forever rein in your heart.

9. What you see as real is an illusion.
    What you see as an illusion is real.

    Visionaries are great at forming ideas in
    the spiritual realm and realizing what
    they have envisioned in the material

world. The spiritual realm, therefore, is the real world where real ideas are born, while the material world is only an illusion. Take that leap of faith based on a dream you have and you will be surprised how attainable it is in the material world.

10. The more negativity I face, the more opportunities I have.

Negativity is simply messages from the Universe steering us in a different direction so we can reach our final destination. This is like the lab mouse in the maze trying to get to the cheese. The mouse always overcomes the blocks in the maze to reach the cheese. Our blocks are mostly emotional and can be overcome through willpower and focus.

11. Free will derails us. Submitting to the plan saves us.

We are given the freedom to choose but not the freedom to deviate from the grand plan. Choose wisely or suffer the consequences. Stay on your path and enjoy success. We are all born to serve a specific function in the mosaic of life, free will therefore is redundant.

12. Swim with the tide, not against it.

Always go with the flow and never against it. The flow may be a new trend that opposes the old trend; thereby creating a new direction. Vacuums are great opportunity creators; knowing in which new direction the tide is headed, is your blessing.

13. Know your role in life and play it well.

Identify your set of skills and resources and apply yourself accordingly into your life path. Train yourself in all that is conducive to you reaching the goal that is compatible with your natural abilities.

14. Follow your life script and forever in heaven you will dwell.

    Only when we are fulfilling our life purpose by being true to our nature is when we are happiest and filled with joy.

15. Which piece of the puzzle of life are you?

    Find out what your function in life is. Become the chef, the engineer, the scientist or any piece of the life puzzle that you were born to be. Being anything else will be tormenting.

16. Know your place in the big picture paradigm.

    We are all here for a reason. It is to create and expand the universe through the use of conditions and resources we were given to accomplish our mission. We are simple contributors to the food chain.

17. Clarity of vision comes from clarity of purpose.

    Once you know your final destination, you will know exactly how to get there despite all the challenges ahead.

18. Life is never what you thought it would be.

    Our life purpose always unfolds in the most mysterious ways and it is never cut and dried as we'd like it to be. It brings out our untapped potential and unveils latent skills we never thought we had.

19. The simpler the better. If it is too complicated, steer clear.

    When things are too complicated, they may be loaded with problems. Why add more problems to your existing pile of problems and make life miserable. Finding stress-free situations on the other hand may prove to be elusive. Your goal, however, is to minimize the presence of stress in your life so as to enjoy a better quality of living.

20. Red flags are a sign from hell. Green flags are a sign from heaven.

Many do not pay attention to the important preview of the movie that is about to be shown. If you are seeing too many bad omens then your movie will end badly. Conversely, if you see too many good omens then chances are your movie will end well. Always be aware of the different messages the Universe sends your way.

21. Luck happens when you are in synch with your natural path.

What better than everything falling into place for you like magic. Many call it luck. I call it "our natural path". The more aligned we are with our true selves, the luckier we are. Luck is the Universe confirming that you are in your element and pursuing the right thing: Lack of luck results from misalignment with our real purpose.

22. Don't try to be a hero, just go with the obvious.

   Why reinvent the wheel when it works well. Many of us attempt to become the superheroes we admire from the comics by trying to reinvent the wheel. Keep it simple and life will become a lot less complicated.

23. The closer you get to your purpose, the more distractions will come your way to derail you.

   This is actually a sign that you are pursuing the right thing. The forces of negativity understand your progress and will make one final big push to steer you off course. It is critical to remain committed.

24. Conquer you fear through focused willpower, and you will conquer defeat.

   The real test of willpower always comes in the form of fear. Commitment is fear's worst nightmare. No committed person is easily swayed by fear.

25. Build your own personal myth and you will be building a solid wall of confidence around you.

Our personal myth stems from our sense of purpose. It is what empowers us to meet and overcome all challenges ahead.

For example, I am great at what I do. I am the best teacher/musician/doctor there is.

26. The more the crowd thinks you are abnormal, the more unique your life purpose is.

Never pay attention to what others feel or think about your plans. Trust only what is within you. Only you can relate to you. Don't rely on others to empathize.

27. Those who dare were born to dare.

    Risk takers promote change, and change is what progress desperately needs in order for humanity to keep forward. They fill their purpose by rattling the status quo and moving us out of our comfort zone.

28. Prophets are innovators and not any more sacred than the rest of us.

    All entrepreneurs are prophets. Be they religious leaders, scientists, business visionaries, philosophers, musicians and so on. They are all inspired by the same Source and cause big changes in their respective fields.

29. Anyone with a noble sense of purpose is a prophet. Stop worshipping other prophets and start honoring yours.

    When you find out what your life purpose is, you will realize that you too are on a mission from the Divine regardless of its magnitude. Focusing on your mission is where your true salvation lies.

30. When you are properly aligned with your purpose, you will come into immense personal power.

When we are finally in our element, we will exude incredible confidence. It will mostly stem from having a set goal to achieve. Having a goal gives us the opportunity to create and become one with the Divine.

II

Personal

1. Become anxious over nothing.

   Detach yourself and have no expectations. If things do not work out then you won't be disappointed. If they do work out, then you will be surprised.

2. Fear nothing and struggle will elude you. Fear everything and anxiety will rule you.

   Fear is mostly baseless and is an invention of the ego. Ninety per cent of what we fear never comes to pass so why worry. Submit yourself to the master plan and release anxiety. What is meant to be is meant to be.

3. The more we try to control, the less we actually have.

   Negative energy can only be repelled with positive. Using negative energy will only exacerbate the problem. Let go and what you are trying to control will be drawn to you. Using more control can only push it further away from you.

4. Avoid excesses and attain inner peace, or dwell on imbalances and face misery.

    All forms of imbalances are destructive and excesses are no different. Excesses lead to volatility and instability. Instability prevents peace from filling your heart.

5. No one punishes or rewards you but you.

    By carefully re-examining all of your successes and failures, you will realize that they are all your own doing. It takes courage to admit one's mistakes and as much courage to admit one's glory.

6. Stick to the plan and enjoy the fruits. Follow your whims and end up in the abyss.

   Maintain discipline in all of your pursuits, and you will be rewarded accordingly. Acting on impulse can only shake such discipline and lead you to deviate from the plan.

7. Choose reason over emotion.

   Let your mind rule your decision-making and never your heart. The heart can be incorporated into the process as long as it doesn't take precedence over the mind.

8. Many of our fears come from guilt.

   We have been conditioned from our early childhood not to go against the rules. Once we do, punishment awaits us; creating fear.

   This little incident, as trivial as it may seem, remains with us in our subconscious, causing many of our emotional blockages. Eliminate the guilt from breaking the rules and you can eliminate many of your fears.

9. Forgive and trust yourself and the world will forgive and trust you.

When we are in a healthy relationship with ourselves i.e. self-respect and confidence, the world will feed us back that same sense of respect and confidence.

Forgiving yourself helps you eliminate much of your guilt and regain love for yourself. When you love and respect yourself, trusting becomes easy.

10. You rule your own universe; therefore, you are responsible for what happens in it.

When your house is in order, all goes according to plan. When it is not, chaos takes over. Ensuring that your house is in order is your responsibility. Blaming others for the chaos in your life only serves as an excuse for the mistakes you have made.

11. Know who and what you are.

Many spend their whole lifetime in darkness not knowing and understanding who they are and what their purpose is. Awaken yourselves and seek the truth out. It will set you free.

12. Who needs the Joneses when you are happy and love who and what you are.

If you had all the treasures of the world, would you look at somebody else's?

Real treasure is found within and is not located in material possessions. When you are happy within, you stand confidently among the crowd where everyone wants to emulate, you instead of you emulating them. By not being comfortable with yourself, you will be emulating others.

13. Boasting is inner weakness. Humility is inner strength.

    When someone is used to and knows success, they do not need to brag about it to the world. Constantly talking about one's success is either exaggeration or fabrication. It is the ego's way of covering up a deeper sense of inadequacy.

14. Forgiving is true power.

    It takes much courage and audacity to let go of the past, no matter how hurtful. It takes even more courage to forgive those who inflicted painful memories on you. By forgiving and forgetting, we let go of the past and move on, otherwise forever remain tormented by the events.

15. Punish not by force but by explaining the lesson behind the punishment.

    Since punishment is sometimes needed to teach lessons, it should not be done in a demeaning way. One should carefully explain what is to be learned from it and leave it in the past. Lessons are needed for us to further evolve.

16. Many of our problems are self-inflicted.

A lot of our problems come from impulsive action without further consideration of possible consequences. Such impulsive action is usually the product of cravings by the five senses and weak self-discipline. Yoga and Tai Chi could greatly help improving those.

17. Keep seeing yourself as the victim and further victimization will come your way.

Ask and you shall receive. Send the message that you are a victim and people will victimize you even more. All the events in your life are a reflection of how you perceive and treat yourself. The kinds of vibes you emit to the universe are the kind that will boomerang back to you.

18. Insecurity craves control. Inner peace relinquishes it.

    Wanting control stems from the constant need for reassurances due to lack of trust. Having full trust, on the other hand, releases that desperate need for reassurances.

19. When we are first honest with ourselves, we can be honest about everything else.

    An honest person is someone who is true to themselves first; someone with enough audacity to admit their wrong doings and is open to solving their problems. Those who continue to live behind false masks are lying to themselves before lying to the rest of the world.

20. It takes courage to admit one's faults and more courage to try to fix or learn from them.

Successful happy people are those who have no problems sharing their faults with the rest of us. It is usually a big indicator that these faults have already been overcome with confidence and; their lessons are retained. Others who hide such faults are mired in deep insecurities, which may also indicate that their lessons were never understood.

21. Focus on the Big Picture and all your suffering will fade.

By not seeing the reason behind your negative event, your suffering will never end. Always try to understand why things did not go as planned and visualize where it is all leading you. Your final destination or big picture may be much better than what you had thought it to be.

22. We all create our own successes and failures.

    When you are well prepared for your exam, passing it becomes highly possible. Treat it lightly and your odds in failing become very real. Combine preparation with proper time and place and winning is surely now at hand.

23. Master your ego and you will master your surroundings.

    Your ego is the source of all negative thoughts and emotions. When it controls you, you view everything as impossible. When you control it, your opportunities abound and the impossible becomes possible. Master your ego by mastering the art of meditation and grounding.

24. Ego is not only arrogance. It is every negative emotion, including fear and self-doubt.

    There's great confusion about what the ego represents and many associate it with arrogance and conceit. Ego is also responsible for all emotions related to the illusion of life such as fear and self-doubt. All of these emotions are limitations the ego creates to hinder our progress. Our greatest challenge on earth is how to subdue our ego so as to realize our earthly dreams.

25. Fear and lack of trust come from within. When we learn how to love and trust ourselves, fear will vanish.

   Fear is the result of past and present traumas that ends up blocking much of our untapped potential. By healing these traumas, one can also heal all fear associated with them.

26. Honesty is not the best policy; self-honesty is.

   In order to be honest with others, one has to be honest with themselves first. Self-honesty is the process of open discussion that one can have with their soul about all the wrong things in their lives, and what can be done to fix them. Such process is always ongoing and never ends since our challenges are a natural component of our daily lives.

27. Balance is key to inner peace.

All can be well when there's harmony between your soul and your physical existence. To reach such a state, one needs to align themselves with their spiritual sense of purpose and live a life of content and acceptance.

28. The balance between logic and emotion is our only salvation.

As both reasonable and emotional beings, it is best that our decisions are based on a good combination between the two. Employing reason for the most part safeguards optimal results.

29. Aim high and expect nothing, you will then receive everything.

The moment we overestimate an outcome, we expose ourselves to disappointment if it falls short. It is however necessary to try our best but more necessary to detach from how it may turn out. By not focusing on the result, you end up perfecting the process, thus producing a better than expected outcome.

30. Duality is life; get used to it.

All things in nature contain light and darkness. Beware of focusing only on one aspect and disregarding the other. It is crucial to note that some may have more of one than the other. Duality is real and necessary for life to thrive.

31. All things in nature have both light and darkness.

Depending on which side you are nurturing deep within you is what you will see in others. Most suspicious people see darkness in others because it is what they see in themselves. Seeing light on the other hand, is a reflection of all the good they see in themselves.

32. Overdoing anything is depreciating its actual value.

The more you love doing something and do it on a day-to-day basis, the closer you will get to disliking it. Doing it in moderation however will always keep that flare for it alive.

33. Excess is deficiency's twin brother. They are both bad for you.

Having too much of something creates disdain for it and having too little creates cravings for it. In both cases, emotions are extreme and extremism in any shape or form is indicative of lack of balance.

34. What you want is not necessarily what you need.

Desire is usually ego driven and what you are wanting may not be what serves you best. Unless it is filling a need that will contribute to a healthy life path, desire should be contained.

35. What you wish for is not necessarily what is best for you.

If your prayers don't come true, then maybe the Universe is asking you to change direction or re-examine your priorities. It is only in our best interest when things flow and not stagnate.

36. Common sense is a rare commodity. Make sure you use it.

All of us have it and very few use it. If we carefully look closer at our daily lives and the mistakes we have made, we realize how absent our common sense is. It is a great tool for avoiding bad decisions.

37. Stand up for yourself no matter what. Respect is earned and not easily given.

   Never give out privileges unless warranted. Humans have this nasty habit of abusing them. Those who do abuse them are showing you how much respect they have for you. Make sure you always draw the line in the sand when needed in order to avoid continued abuse.

38. Profanity is character in decline

   Using lots of profanity is indicative of decline in self-restrain and discipline. Such language contains negative energy and is indicative of serious personal crisis.

39. Promote self-discipline and you will elevate self-esteem.

   Being disciplined is a sign of sound personal structure and organization. When these are present, your decisions are most likely well-calculated and properly balanced. This leads to confidence and a higher self-image.

40. Your language is the mirror of your true self-worth. Choose your words carefully.

The words you use to describe others or situations are a reflection of how you perceive yourself. By calling someone an idiot, you are inferring that you are the idiot. Refraining from using any negative words implies self-respect.

III

Progress

1. All without exception is subject to evolution. Nothing is etched in stone including Divine revelation.

   Let's be honest with ourselves and examine ancient writings and life in general. Evolution is real; otherwise we would all be having dinner with dinosaurs today. Ancient writings have many great things to say, but a lot of it has been frozen in time and needs severe overhauling so as to bring it into our current century. The Creator invented evolution for a reason. That reason is progress.

2. Knowledge is empowerment. Lack of it is enslavement.

   When you know the answers, you cannot be fooled or controlled. When you don't, anyone can have control over you. Free yourself through knowledge.

3. Limiting is human. Infinite is Divine.

    When you connect to your spiritual self, all you would see is the infinite possibilities. When you are confined to your human self, all you would dwell on is scarcity.

4. Knowledge is expansive. Ignorance is constricting.

    When you are constantly seeking knowledge, your horizons naturally expand. When you don't know much about anything, the earth will always seem flat.

5. Never assume or judge. Always explore and trust.

    Assumption is the mother of all mishaps. By assuming, we undermine. By undermining, we make mistakes. If you think you know it all, then chances are you know nothing. Venture out and learn. This is how you expand your possibilities and can start trusting. How can you trust anything you have not explored or researched?

6. Sticking to one perspective is spiritual and intellectual suicide.

This is like going to a court system with only the judge to produce the verdict without any help from the jury. If only one judge possesses the truth, then the truth is limited.

Follow that single truth blindly and you will be giving away your personal power.

7. Refrain from asking questions and delay your evolution.

The more questions we ask, the more knowledge we acquire. Knowledge is key to helping us move up to our next evolutionary stage. Stop asking questions and you will forever remain stagnant.

8. Challenges are lessons and are not evil.

   All negative events are opportunities for us to learn lessons so we can grow and evolve. Imagine going through school without any exams. How much would you learn?

   By embracing these events as blessings in disguise, we solidify our resolve to living a meaningful life.

9. They who know history can predict the future.

   By knowing and understanding past patterns, we are able to predict how it will all unfold in the future. Although the only thing constant in the universe is change, the laws of physics are almost always the same. History always repeats itself due to recurring patterns in nature. Study past patterns and you could predict future ones.

10. Applying old solutions to new problems is utter madness.

    What worked in the past may no longer be feasible in the present due to changing circumstances and conditions. The world is ever evolving, and unless we adapt our ways, we will fall behind. Sticking to old fundamentals in any shape or form is a recipe for disaster.

11. All imbalances will eventually be rectified.

    Always be wary when imbalances are occurring. It may take long time, but the equation will even out. If you see imbalances, then rest assured that a correction is coming. The laws of physics have to always even out.

12. The more we learn, the more we need to learn.

    Since knowledge is infinitely expansive, learning seems to be as limitless as the universe itself. All new discoveries are followed by newer discoveries that seem endless.

13. Learning about the Infinite is infinitely without limits.

   No one human could explain it all since all is ad infinitum. An infinite amount of teachers could try, but they will still fall short since this whole process is endless.

14. There is no single answer. There is an infinite number of answers.

   Everyone professes their version of the truth; as long as they don't claim to be the only conveyors of it. Their version may appeal to some but never everyone. This is what makes the diversity of creation so amazing.

15. Evolve or die. It is your choice to make.

   By limiting your own progress, you hinder your evolution. When evolution ends, life becomes pointless unless you willingly choose to remain in junior high for the rest of your life.

16. Death is not only physical. It could also be intellectual and spiritual.

   When we are spiritually hollow, our ability to focus may weaken, and it starts feeling like living in this world but not of this world.

IV

Relationships

1. Love at first sight is similar to crash and burn.

   As fast as anything rises, it will fall. Therefore, it is best to avoid crazy adrenaline-based love and look for something more gradual and stable.

2. If they care enough, they will handle you with care.

   Do not fall for excuses and expect absolute care. Ask yourself how you would have handled it if you truly cared. Always put yourself in other's shoes and see what answers you come up with.

3. Not returning calls or messages indicates apathy or lack of respect.

   Would you have made the effort to call back if you truly cared about the person?

4. People do not play games. They are either interested or have other agendas.

   Hesitation or lack of interest is what produces the perception of playing games. When one is interested, all barriers come down and honesty and openness become the norm.

5. Infatuation is a recipe for disaster.

   When one is infatuated, they are blinded by emotion and misguided by chemical reactions. Take a deep breath and regain your sanity before digging a deeper hole.

6. Fall in love with yourself and others will fall in love with you.

   You attract those who are like you. If you fear commitment then you will attract those who do not want to commit. If you dislike yourself then you will be drawn to those with negative self-image. Only when you love yourself is when you will attract those with a healthy self-esteem.

7. Love is capable of producing hate.

    Emotions are tricky things and should never be tampered with. When emotions are in control, they can swing from one extreme to another. The more intense the emotion, the deeper the reaction is.

8. Using shallow means to attract love is a sign of low self-esteem.

    Anyone exploiting the five senses to attract love is covering up for deficiencies in character and/or intellect. Similarly, those who are attracted by such means see very little value in substance.

9. When relationships are lacking in mutual respect, their viability becomes questionable.

   Boundaries are the necessary evil for those who do not respect you. No one with self-respect should allow others to cross them. The more you refrain from erecting boundaries, the more abuse you will face.

10. Look for character and you will find stability.

    Character is the basic foundation of one's personality. Focus on finding solid character and you will have a healthy relationship. When you focus on superficial traits such as looks, money, and sex you will end up with a relationship founded on shaky grounds.

11. Slowly evolving love lasts. Instant love fades.

   True love grows on the backs of struggle, sacrifice and many lessons a couple endures together. Overcoming these lessons is what helps grow a solid foundation for any relationship.

12. Find those who balance you and not who are similar to you.

   A body cannot have two heads. Shoulders are just as important so the head can lay on the body. If you are a driver in the relationship then you will need to find a passenger. Finding another driver will only send the car in two different directions, which ultimately will lead the relationship to nowhere.

13. If you are second guessing, move on.

   When in doubt, do absolutely nothing. Your mind, body, and soul have to all be aligned in confirming what you are considering. When you spend too much time thinking about someone or something, it may not be part of your natural path.

14. It is not about money, sex, appearance, religion, race, or politics. It's about character.

    Stop looking for all the wrong reasons on why you should like someone. Character is the criteria upon which solid foundation is built. Anything else yields nothing but short term gains.

15. To make it through thick and thin, you need harmony.

    To overcome challenges, a couple would have to be in complete synch with one another and form a cohesive unit to go to battle every day and win.

16. Fear of being alone is not warranted.
    Fear of being abused is.

    If one is afraid of being alone then one is
    not at peace. When you love the person
    within, you won't mind spending all the
    time in the world with them. Many stay
    in bad relationships out of fear of being
    alone. One cannot solve a problem by
    taking on more problems.

17. No one abuses anyone without their
    permission.

    The moment this starts happening,
    you should instantly put an end to it;
    otherwise you end up issuing an open
    invitation to its repetition. No self-
    respecting individual would allow that
    to continue.

18. Flattery keeps it all alive. Constant
    comforting does too.

    Make sure to always give compliments
    out and provide a sense of security;
    they create an atmosphere of positivity

and appreciation. This in turn will feed you back true love and support.

19. Always give and take.

Whenever you take without giving back, you risk creating imbalances that lead to resentment. Always try to give back so everyone feels they are treated fairly.

20. The grass is greener only in a galaxy far, far away.

This is one of the major signs that we are starting to take things for granted and losing appreciation for what you have. The grass appears greener only when we have stability in our lives; and thus start looking for excitement. Once we get to the other side, however, we will realize how faded the grass actually is.

21. If they are too hot to handle then chances are you will get burned.

    Beware of those who think too highly of themselves. They may see you as irrelevant to their lives. Always avoid the overvalued and go with the fairly valued.

22. Know yourself first and those who know what they want will come knocking on your door.

    When you understand what works and does not work for you, those who understand the same about themselves will show up in your life.

23. Breaking hearts is like breaking glass. Once the damage is done, gluing the pieces back together is almost impossible.

    Emotional hurt is the worst kind since it is unpredictable and could have disastrous consequences. Many could forgive but few would completely forget.

24. Masks do not survive the honeymoon.

   True colors take three to six months on average to surface. Once the passion settles down, all masks start coming off.

25. Be real, right from the start and you will avoid disappointment later on.

   Put all of your cards on the table right from the beginning and ask them to do the same, this way no unrealistic expectations are made.

26. If someone is not open then they are hiding something.

   Anyone keeping secrets has an agenda. It could also be due to serious trust issues or lack of confidence in whatever they are proposing.

27. I t is not worth saving unless it adds value to your life.

Sometimes you just have to be honest with yourself and cut your losses while you can. When someone does not treat you right or add value to your life, it is best to let them go. This is not to suggest utility at all. There are those worth the sacrifice since they honor you the way you would honor yourself.

28. Everyone is a nice person but not everyone balances you.

There are many great people out there but very few 'right ones' for you. The right ones are those who complement you and not turn your life into a constant boxing match. Energies have got to always flow for all to be well.

V

Religion

1. Believing in and following only one spiritual path is placing limitations on the soul's full potential. This is like choosing to eat only one type of cuisine all of your life while missing out on the delights and benefits of all the others.

   Explore what others have to say. You would be surprised how much you can learn from them and how it would help improve your quality of life.

2. Diversity in all shapes and forms is the Creator's gift to the world. It should all therefore be embraced and celebrated since it emanates from the same sacred source.

   Imagine how boring and limiting if we had no variety in life. All was created to serve a purpose, and each and every creation has certain uniqueness to it. Diversity is what helps us grow by learning from each other.

3. What a disservice to the Creator it is to not believe in or explore the impossible.

    Anyone claiming to "not believe" is expressing lack of faith in their personal full potential. This may stem from deeply embedded insecurities and a need to remain dormant in their comfort zone. Time and time again it has been proven that the impossible is very possible. The Infinite is called the Infinite for a reason-without any limitations.

4. Stop worshiping the messenger; start applying the message.

    Those who follow teachings blindly are not aware of the actual teachings; and more inclined towards worshiping the teacher. By worshiping the teacher, they fill a desperate need for a savior to come and salvage them from their misery. They fail to realize that their salvation lies in taking charge and applying the teachings instead of worshiping the teacher. We are all our own saviors. Teachers are only here to provide guidance.

5. If God is the Infinite then no one single human teacher could explain it all. It would require an infinite number of teachers to arrive at the truth.

    There are no special teachers and they all have something important to say. Although they should be greatly admired for their guidance, one should carefully scrutinize everything they have said and never take it out of context. Some teachings survive the passage of time, but not all of them do.

6. Assuming to know it all is assuming to be on equal footing with the Infinite.

    Only the Infinite knows what the Infinite has created, therefore no human can conceptualize what is truly out there. This is why it is important to remain open to all possibilities.

7. Claiming to have access to the truth
    is claiming to have the ability to read
    the Infinite's mind.

    Self-righteousness is the kiss of death.
    It stops people short of their true
    potential by assuming they know it all,
    since they believe to be in possession of
    the mythical Holy Grail.

8. Stop following humans and start
    listening to your Divine self.

    We all have the ability to inspire
    ourselves by eliminating much of what
    is blocking us. It takes faith and courage
    to reach that state of self-honesty and
    start deleting all the toxic memories
    and emotions, needed to recreate our
    lives.

9. Why connect to the Infinite through
    others when we can directly do it
    ourselves.

    By cleaning up our emotional toxicity,
    we avail room for Divine inspiration to

flow in and help create our new selves. No one else can do it for us.

10. Time to eliminate the middle man and go directly to the Source.

   Those promising you eternity by following them are eternally stripping away your personal power and do not want you to reach enlightenment. We are personally responsible for our own awakening. It is redundant to seek it through another human being.

11. No one should suffer for someone else's mistakes. Mistakes are part of our spiritual evolution.

   We are all personally responsible for our own faults, and it is absurd to carry the burden of guilt for somebody else's pain.

12. Ancient dogmas served their purpose. Time to move on.

   Those insisting on ancient systems are living in a world where time has been frozen. Changes in attitude necessitate a change in belief systems. What was revealed previously may prove to be antiquated when applied presently.

13. Dogma is complexity. Reconnecting is simplicity.

   As human society grows in complexity, the need for simplicity arises. Dogma is the unfortunate smothering of our daily existence. It is no longer required to communicate with the Divine. Reconnect spiritually through meditation and maintain simplicity. A simple life is your key to true salvation.

14. Do not fear God. Love Him.

   The days of using fear to instill discipline are gone. Humans today need understanding to appreciate.

When we understand the Divine and His lessons to serve our highest good, we will develop natural love for Him.

15. We worship by creating and not destroying.

    By fulfilling our life purpose of adding value to the universe, we automatically service the Creator. Lighting candles and asking for gifts are not the point. Helping in the creation process is.

16. Faith in us is the same as faith in the Divine. Only when such faith is present, Divine inspiration comes down through us to create.

    If we are lacking faith in ourselves, that may be due to our disconnecting from the Divine. To reconnect, one needs to release much of the negativity blocking such connections from taking place.

17. Lack of faith in us is the same as lack of faith in the Divine. Only when such a void is present, our ability to destroy is manifested.

    It is hard for both light and darkness to occupy the same space. When light is not present, darkness comes in to fill the void, thereby wreaking havoc on your soul.

18. The need to control or destroy is same as the lack of Divinity within.

    Negative tendencies are a product of the dark side and can easily manifest once our connection to the Divine is lost. Control and destroy are two emotions that emanate from a deeper sense of fear and hate.

19. You push first and God will push next as long as you are pushing in the right direction.

    It takes a leap of faith to make dramatic changes to your life. But without you initiating the first step, the Divine will not step in to help. The Universe will only step in after you have set a powerful intention to move ahead. Just make sure that you only move forward after confirming your life purpose, otherwise the Divine will not step in.

20. Manifesting lies in the delicate balance between prayer and action.

Prayer is the soul searching that is required prior to taking action. At the end of the day, a combination of the two is what manifests miracles, and leads you to realizing your dreams.

21. Prayer is the attempt to communicate with God. Meditation is directly connecting with Him.

Prayer is asking the Heavens for things to materialize, while meditation enables you to receive instant answers on how to make things work.

22. Heaven and hell are within. We experience one or the other depending on decisions we make.

    The number of blessings or curses in our lives is direct evidence of how well or poorly we have chosen. Follow the rules of sanity and sanity will find you. Follow those of insanity and insanity will engulf you.

23. Karma is necessary for our evolution. One lifetime is not enough to complete all of our karmas.

    If the soul is to keep on evolving and reach perfection, then one lifetime is surely not enough to learn all required lessons. Reincarnation is the different stages of evolution the soul has to climb in order to reach divinity.

24. Enlightenment is the near completion of karma.

    When the soul has accumulated enough lessons and is nearing perfection, it is said to be enlightened. Enlightenment is the stage of knowing when you just know that you know and no one else can relate but you.

25. Those who do not understand have few more karmas to complete.

The knowing happens when there is no more knowing to be had. This is when all lessons have been completed and the time to teach is upon you.

26. Those seeking the truth are upon enlightenment.

Those looking to "know" are closest to the truth than the rest of all of us. It is then when one is no longer veiled from God.

27. The truth is subjective and never objective. This is why there are infinite versions of it.

    There are many visions, many perspectives and many proclaiming themselves to be prophets and messiahs; this is according to whom?

    Beware of those preaching their divinity when "Servants of the Universe" should be their main title.

28. Good or evil? Glass half full or half empty?

    It's all a matter of perspective depending on which side of the aisle you are seated. The Yin and Yang is perhaps what best describes it.

29. Your evil is someone else's good and your good is someone else's evil. Exceptions do apply.

    Your terrorist is someone else's freedom fighter and your freedom fighter is someone else's terrorist. Who is good and who is evil?

Pedophiles qualify as an exception.

30. It is not God vs. the devil, it is stability vs. thrill.

Stability seldom leads to trouble while excitement thrives on it. Pursue things that are of a stable nature and you will avoid anxiety. Seek thrill continuously, and you will live under constant stress.

31. God is not a dictator, so stop presenting Him as one.

The old ways of using fear and guilt are over. There's a new God in town and He is forgiving and loving. Understand His lessons and you will understand His love for you.

32. It does not matter how much you pray for something to happen. What matters is whether it is for your highest good or not.

    Before asking for gifts from the Heavens, start focusing on whether they serve your best interest or not. Your highest good is always on His mind.

33. Beware of those offering you the keys to paradise, for they most likely reside in hell.

    Paradise is a state of mind and not a piece of real estate. Such state is attainable through personal empowerment and not subjected to somebody else's agenda.

34. Be wary of those promising to bring you salvation through their deities. The only one capable of saving your soul is you.

    True salvation lies within and not without. When we are finally and consciously ready to change our lives, solutions will surface and our road to healing our spirit begins.

VI

Politics

1. Dictatorships enslave by force. Democracies enslave by choice.

   Dictatorships use the secret service to instill fear in the masses so as to control them. Democracies use the media to extract our full submission to the system through influencing choices we deliberately make.

2. The underdog counts the most, not the dog.

   Since the underdog represents the majority, they hold the key to stability. The elite needs the masses more than the masses need the elite. Although, ultimately a good balance between the two is what is necessary for the health of any system.

3. Leadership comes from within.

   The values of a society get passed on to its leaders. If a society is selfish, then more likely its leadership will be selfish. If a society is disciplined then so is its leadership. Blaming problems on leadership is then absurd. A society needs to look within for sources of its problems.

4. Share and prosper or hoard and struggle.

    No one could prosper single handedly. We all do it through the help of others along the way. It is critical then to share our success with those who helped us attain it. Failing to do so, would result in losing support and eluding prosperity.

5. What serves the few is not sustainable. What serves the many is forever lasting.

    Systems prosper by strengthening their middle class and not their elite. History is filled with examples of the average revolting against the unfair elite. The elite may be able to support injustice for as long as the middle man is dormant. Once awakened, the middle man will impose change. By keeping it fair, the stability of the system would last indefinitely.

6. Govern by the people, for the people; and not by the privileged, for the privileged.

    When the people own it and feel it is theirs, they will treat it with care. For a society to respect its government, the government has to serve everyone and not only those with "access".

7. Cater to the people and they will believe.

    People are led by fulfilled promises and not empty ones. Show them positive results and they will become your support system.

8. Fear not the awakened, but those who are asleep, for one day they will also be awakened.

   The bigger the number of those who are asleep, the bigger their impact will be once enlightened. We are seeing current examples of this in Egypt, Libya, and Russia.

9. Treat with fairness and forever reign in your kingdom.

   You are appointed by the people and they are who you answer to. To keep your job as ruler, you will need to maintain a fair system of governance. You are respected as a public servant through your deeds and not empty words.

10. Serve humbly those who chose you to serve them, and immortality is yours to keep.

    People seem to always forgive and forget those who mistreat them but never forget those who were kind to them. Saddam

Hussein or Stalin's monuments are no longer standing while Lincoln's and many others still are.

11. Nations are as powerful as their value system is. When values weaken, so do nations.

A good governing system could only work if the discipline behind it is present. Discipline comes from a solid value system and strict adherence to ethical principles.

12. Pragmatism works. Rigidity doesn't.

The flexibility of any system is what ultimately makes it work. Flexibility is incorporating the various variables of life into a system, normally overlooked by theory. Rigidity is sticking to theory and ignoring the existence of such variables, which may prove to be detrimental.

13. A nation is as obsolete as its system is.

   Nations who dwell on antiquated dogmas are stuck in a glorious past that will never make a comeback. Illusions of returning to such a past can only be healed by subduing the national ego and proper education. Everyone gets their turn in history. Accept it and move on.

14. To make history, a nation needs to learn from the past.

   By examining trials and errors of previous great nations, a nation can help avoid many of its shortcomings. Time is a nation's best ally if utilized properly.

15. A great nation that needs an enemy to justify its *raison d'être* is one that is in decline.

   A great nation is one upon which the world is dependent for produced goods and services, as well as inventions serving mankind. It is not one whose sole purpose is to provide protection from a certain enemy.

16. Ascending nations are those who care very little about politics and more about building wealth.

Rising powers understand the need to accumulate wealth first in order to build up their military. Their business-as-usual attitude and avoiding costly wars are what end up helping them reach new heights.

17. A Democratic civilization is one that has reached its peak and whose decline is around the corner.

Democracy signals the height of a civilization and it usually stems from the rise of an affluent middle class demanding more say in the political process. No civilization starts out democratically.

18. Pity the nation whose main concern is bread and circuses.

A nation pre-occupied primarily with fun and games is one on the verge of losing its competitive edge and is more than likely headed towards bankruptcy.

19. Nations, who use fear to control their masses, are bankrupt regarding new ideas.

When ideas on how to create new economic opportunity run out, fear becomes the best means of controlling the frustration of the people.

20. Empire is the beginning of the end of a great civilization.

Empire is the ultimate stage of a civilization and usually implies peak. The question then arises on how much longer, can such a peak last.

21. When the pyramid has been flattened out, chaos ensues.

    Healthy structures are pyramid-like and consist of a tip, the middle and the base. When all three tiers become one level, structure is no longer present and chaos is to follow. We see it, for example, in how children today no longer fear parental authority.

22. When values become twisted, the death spiral has begun.

    When permissiveness becomes the norm and traditions are overturned, a social and moral crisis is at hand; leading into the abyss.

23. Equality is a myth. Sharing access is not.

    We are all equal in value but never in competencies. This is no excuse, however, to not have equal access to available resources.

24. Too much equality is no equality at all.

    When you give too much of anything to anyone, its value no longer holds. By giving too many rights to a particular group, you will inevitably infringe on the rights of another group.

25. A society with too much crime is lacking in justice.

    When justice is always rightly served, many will believe in and respect the judicial system. The presence of too much crime in a society is indicative of a judicial system that is lacking in credibility.

26. Laws should be enacted to serve the majority and not the exception.

    What is good for the whole should also be good for the few, but what is good for the few is not always good for the whole. Some may have to sacrifice so the majority can benefit.

27. A good leader is one who is bold and blunt enough to tell the truth regardless of political consequences.

True leadership is about doing the right thing and not what helps in the election process. Those fearing political consequences have nothing to fear. The people appreciate honesty and boldness.

28. In order to make peace, one has to be open to compromise and be ready to forgive and forget.

Peace is as elusive as the negotiating parties like it to be. Only when a genuine intent of reaching an agreement is present, prior to the negotiations, peace can be achieved. Anything else is fog.

29. Individualism destroys the fabric of a nation. Self-responsibility builds it.

    Individualism leads to lack of cohesiveness and the rise in selfish behavior. Self-responsibility accounts for all actions and produces a fundamentally sound society.

30. When children learn their values from other children, it's all downhill from there.

    Values are the building blocks of a society. They must be properly instilled in children by their parents in order for them to have a healthy future. Children teaching children values, is similar to the blind leading the blind.

31. Nations fall only when they have already fallen from within.

    When a nation is fundamentally strong, no enemy can defeat it. Defeat always comes on the backs of weak fundamentals, such as, deteriorating values and lack of trust in its governing system.

32. Confident systems have no use for scapegoats, fragile ones do.

Using the blame game to push away responsibility for failure is a sign of weakness. A confident nation always assumes responsibility and tries to solve its problems on its own.

VII

Finances

1. Live frugally and eliminate unease. Spend frivolously and suffer the consequences.

   What is better than living within your means and going to sleep at night knowing all of your bills are easily paid? Anything different will exert pressure on you and bring about anxiety and lack of sleep.

2. It is not the banker's fault. You are the one to blame.

   Unless you signed the dotted line with a gun pointed to your head, you are solely responsible for your debt woes. Your lack of financial discipline is the culprit here and not your lenders. Be honest with yourself.

3. Spend more than you make! Does that make any sense?

   Balancing your checkbook should be as important as breathing. One cannot breathe properly when overwhelmed by stressful finances.

4. Overspending to please others? Do you really dislike yourself that much?

    Why should you care about how others perceive you when you are in love with who you are? Those living to please others are self-loathing and have no sense of personal independence. They are dependent on someone else's opinion because they don't have favorable ones of themselves.

5. Obsessive materialism is spiritual void.

    Anyone crazed with accumulating material possessions is trying to fill a big void in their spiritual life. When we are spiritually fulfilled, materialistic pursuits become irrelevant.

6. Desire for the material is lack of satisfaction with oneself.

    When we are unhappy inside, we end up buying cars and houses and work extra hours to escape our "inner" reality. Meanwhile, the solution is deep within.

7. Insecurities feed on earthly wants.

    One cannot fill spiritual gaps with material items. Try meditation, grounding and reconnecting to your essence. Your true essence is your link to the Divine where weakness is replaced with strength.

8. When we are inadequate inside, we seek "outside" factors to compensate.

    Some may turn to hedonistic pursuits and/or destructive addictions. They serve as temporary solutions to chronic problems. To solve long term problems, you are better off seeking deeper and more lasting solutions. For that, you would need to address the source of the issue.

9. Focus on serving the universe first, and money will come. Focus on money first, and the universe will abandon you.

    If money is your primary objective, then rest assured your venture won't last long. Serving the universe is what ensures your longevity in the business world.

10. What you are promoting is what counts, not how much it can generate for you.

    Always link your career path to serving mankind and not yourself. Success comes from the ability to fill a need and not a personal agenda to acquire wealth. Wealth is only the result of doing the right thing.

11. Pursue your life purpose and joy will fill your heart. Chase after money all of your life and experience acute sadness.

    When you are doing what comes naturally to you, abundance appears out of nowhere. When you do not do what comes naturally to you, you will continue to struggle financially.

12. Serving the five senses is limiting. Adhering to spiritual law is riveting.

    Decisions based on gratifying materialistic desires produces short term gains, whereas basing it on spiritual values produces sound long term results.

13. Why embrace stress when you could be living at ease.

    It's a simple straight forward answer, yet many choose to embrace stress. When pursuing what is naturally yours, stress is contained, otherwise it runs amuck.

14. Cars and homes don't make you. Character does.

   Although superficiality sells, its gains are short-lived. Many of us unfortunately are taken by what is on the surface rather than looking beneath it. Always focus on fundamentals and you will see through the illusion.

15. The piper always shows up to collect. Do not believe you're special.

   Delays may happen, but the inevitable always arrives. There are always consequences to pay and no one is immune. We have seen it time and time again. For every action there is always a reaction.

16. If it is too easy to acquire, it will be easier to lose.

    No one gets there without paying their dues. Dues are what make us appreciate how we got there. When we don't struggle to get it, we will not fight to keep it.

17. Earn it and you will preserve it. Do not earn it and you will most definitely waste it.

    When it is given to us, we will not hold onto it with our dear lives. We will appreciate it a lot more if we have to struggle for it. When it's taken for granted, we will not understand its actual value and end up giving it away.

18. Beware of free lunches; they never sit well with you.

    There are always consequences no matter what. Do not be fooled by those offering you the moon and expecting nothing in return. For every winner out there, there's a loser. No one would be giving anything away unless they have some kind of vested interest in the process. Even when charities give away to the poor, they would have to take it from philanthropists who feel the urge to give back.

19. There are no guarantees in life; except for death.

    All is subject to speculation and forecast, otherwise there is no point in taking risk. Calculated risk does exist; all it does is minimize the odds against you. Looking for assurances is like asking for the answers to the exam's questions without having to study for it.

20. Whoever promises guarantees is preaching death.

    No one knows the future and nothing is ever etched in stone. We have the ability to alter the future by always changing paths. For anyone to come out and offer future certainties, is most likely talking about death, because it is the only thing in life that is certain.

21. One plus one has to always equal two, otherwise it is time to jump ship.

   If it does not add up, then most likely it is not real. All equations have to check out and when they don't be afraid, be very afraid.

22. Fundamentals always win out. You just need to be patient.

   It may take some time for what is not real to get exposed, but getting exposed is what will happen to it. Anything lacking in substance is not real. Having substance, therefore, should always be your primary reason to invest.

23. It's all about balance sheets. Assets vs. liabilities and nothing more complicated than that.

    You can analyze and overanalyze but at the end of the day, your true worth is determined by the value of the assets you own vs. how much you owe. You can apply this to individuals, businesses and governments.

24. Follow the money trail and stop overanalyzing.

    It could be the most attractive concept on the planet, yet draws absolutely no interest from the general public. What sells is not always logical, but the money behind it may be real. Sticking, however, to fundamentals is what keeps you on the safe side.

25. Analysts are those who think they know and are hoping that you do not know.

   There is always your average performer who does not know much and your star performer who knows a lot. Unfortunately, average performers have a much wider reach than star performers and end up leading many astray. One way to test out their competence is by asking tons of questions and verifying all the answers.

26. To make money, you need to solve a problem.

   Most of our inventions are discovered randomly by trying to find a solution to a problem. Look for vacuums and find out where the next deficiency will be occurring, then try to cover that gap. It is like solving a giant mathematical equation.

27. It's all about filling a need. Nothing more and nothing less.

    Many attempt at wealth creation by all means necessary without paying attention to how they want to create it. Ultimately, it is as simple as finding a gap in the market place and trying to fill it. Gaps are constantly happening before us but we have got to pay attention to how we can exploit them.

28. Saturation is the beginning of decline. Rock bottom is the beginning of ascent.

    Saturation is similar to exhaustion. When exhaustion happens, what follows is rest or collapse. Either way, it is not a good scenario. Rock bottom, on the other hand, is a sign that a rebound is coming and an ascent is now more plausible. Beware, however, that saturation may be the beginning of death and rock bottom may be death itself. It all depends on how intact the overall trend is.

29. Two partners alike have no need for partnership.

   If two partners are bringing the same skills to the table then what good is the partnership? Moreover, two partners possessing the same character is a recipe for disaster.

30. Complement one another in partnership and watch business boom.

   Match your strengths with your partner's weaknesses and their strengths with your weaknesses and you can build yourselves a prosperous business relationship.

   Conflict usually happens when the two are trying to compete in the same arena. Your partner should never be your competition.

31. Jump in when everyone is jumping out and jump out when everyone is jumping in.

It is said that ninety percent of the masses are wrong ninety percent of the time. It is wise then to go against what the masses typically do, rather than go with them. This probably happens because many buy or sell on emotion vs. the few who buy and sell on reason.

32. Fools are those who think that everyone else is a fool.

Cheating the masses may work in the short run, but eventually one of them will wake up and expose the lie herein.

33. For one to prosper, one has to produce and sell, not consume and spend.

Those who manufacture for the world, end up ruling it. Manufacturing produces real goods to sell. Real income is then generated, and with income comes saving and investing, thus leading to prosperity. Consuming on the other hand is the same as spending. No one prospers by basing their existence on spending.

34. Overvalued is not interesting; undervalued is.

Opportunity lies where there's room for growth and not where there's maturity and saturation. Undervalued is still working hard to become overvalued, whereas overvalued no longer needs to work hard at all and is beginning to take it all for granted.

35. You measure the health of an economy with the resilience of its middle class, and not the wealth of its elite.

The middle class is the social, moral and financial backbone of a society. As the middle class goes, so does the rest of the country. Healthy economies are usually three-tiered and contain a prosperous middle class. Impoverished economies are polarized between rich and poor in a two-tiered system.

36. Invest in the people behind the concept, but never the concept alone.

   Although many concepts seem promising enough to invest in, many of them end up failing due to bad management. It takes a solid team of managers and workers to help make any concept succeed.